OTITIS MEDIA

a Pocket Guide

Michael Hawke, M.D.
Professor of Otolaryngology and Pathology
Faculty of Medicine
University of Toronto

Chief, Department of Otolaryngology
St. Joseph's Health Centre
Toronto, Ontario, Canada

Produced by
Decker Periodicals Inc., Hamilton, Canada

Publisher: Isabel Wrotkowski
Design: boyes and connolly
Cover illustration: Leah Stephenson-Aurini
Printed and bound in Canada

CONTENTS

Introduction *v*

1 **Acute Otitis Media** *1*

2 **Casts and Crusts of the Tympanic Membrane** *49*

3 **Mastoiditis** *57*

4 **Mucoid Otitis Media** *64*

5 **Serous Otitis Media** *83*

6 **Indications for Tympanocentesis or Myringotomy** *97*

7 **Tube Granuloma** *111*

8 **Atelectasis of the Middle Ear** *118*

9 **Adhesive Otitis Media** *122*

10 **Cholesteatoma** *125*

11 **Antibiotic Treatment** *127*

Glossary *133*

Index *135*

INTRODUCTION

Apart from well-baby checkups and routine examinations, otitis media is the most common reason children are seen in physicians' offices. This pocket guide has been prepared to assist the practitioner in the diagnosis and management of the patient who presents with otitis media.

This pocket guide was produced
with the assistance of a
generous educational grant from
SmithKline Beecham, Canada

Otitis media is a generic term applied to a series of distinct conditions that, with the exception of serous otitis media, are all characterized by the presence of either inflammation or infection of the mucosal lining of the middle-ear cleft, or by the sequelae of such inflammation. For purposes of clarity, the different types of otitis media are classified in the following table

Clinical Classification of Otitis Media

Type	Synonyms	Abbreviation
Acute Otitis Media	Suppurative Purulent Bacterial	AOM
Mucoid Otitis Media	Otitis Media with Effusion "Glue ear" Secretory Otitis Media	MOM
Serous Otitis Media		SOM
Chronic Suppurative Otitis Media	Chronic Otitis Media	CSOM

ACUTE OTITIS MEDIA

Synonym

- Acute suppurative otitis media

Definition

- An acute bacterial infection of the middle-ear cleft

Symptoms

- Acute onset of severe otalgia (earache)
- Acute onset of hearing loss
- Fever
- Malaise
- Irritability (in infants)
- Pulling at the ear (in infants)
- Gastrointestinal symptoms, vomiting and diarrhea (in infants)

Epidemiology

Age

- Otitis media is predominantly a disease of infants and young children; propensity for the very young to contract the disease is probably due to the differences, between infants and adults, in the length, width, angle and

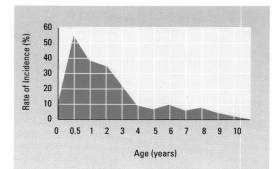

The peak annual incidence rate of 51.6 percent occurs at 6 to 12 months of age, steadily declining thereafter. *Source*: Hilditch JR: *J Otolaryngology* 14(6)366, 1985

consequently the functional competence of the bony eustachian tube

- With each year, the ear develops more resistance to otitis media
- By three years of age, more than two thirds of children have had at least one episode of acute otitis media (AOME), and one third will have had three or more episodes[*]

[*]Teele DW: *Paediatrics* 74(2) 282, 1984

Sex

- Otitis media slightly more common in males; difference is probably due to an overall difference, between the sexes, in the rate of childhood infections

Race

- Increased incidence of otitis media in Eskimos, American Indians and Hispanics
- Increased incidence of otorrhea in Eskimos and American Indians
- Decreased incidence in Blacks
- Differences probably due to variations, amongst ethnic groups, in the length, width and angle of the bony Eustachian tube, and consequently the functional competence of the Eustachian tube in American Blacks, Whites, and Indians

Risk Factors in Acute Otitis Media

Age

- Uncommon in first six months of life
- Most common from age six to 11 months
- Generally more common in the first two years of life
- Children having their first attack of AOM before age one are more prone to recurrent episodes than those children having their first attack after one year of age. The most obvious reason for this peak in incidence is the

relatively low concentration of protective immunoglobulins in the first two years of life, with the exception of the first six months of life, during which the maternal immunoglobulins that have been transmitted through the placenta to the infant provide a significant degree of protection.

Breast Feeding

- Less common in breast-fed children
- Fewer recurrent attacks in breast-fed children

Familial Predisposition

- More common in children with a positive family history of ear infections

Allergy

- Increased incidence in children with an atopic diathesis, e.g., any allergy, including milk allergies, drug allergies, etc.

Minor Immune Deficiency

- Increased incidence in children with repeated upper-respiratory infections
- More common in children with histories of cold in the week prior to onset of AOM
- Children with six or more episodes of AOM are considered to be "otitis-prone"
- Immune status of these children, especially Ig G subclass 2 and 4, should be checked

Seasonal Variation

- Increased incidence during the "cold season," i.e., the winter months, January through March

Housing

- More common in urban areas
- More common in children living in apartments

Day Care

- More common in children attending community day-care centers
- More persistent in children attending community day-care centers
- More common in children attending larger (more than 10 children) day-care centers

Environmental Factors

- More common in infants who have humidifiers in their bedrooms

Pathogenesis

- Acute otitis media is the result of a bacterial infection, by pathogenic bacteria, of the middle-ear cleft
- Mucosal lining of the middle-ear cleft is especially vulnerable to the retrograde spread of

infection from the upper-respiratory tract
- Organisms causing the infection enter the middle-ear cleft from the nasopharynx, via the Eustachian tube

The Role of the Eustachian Tube in the Pathogenesis of Acute Otitis Media

- The Eustachian tube in infants and young children is:
  - short
  - allows reflux from the nasopharynx into the middle ear
  - has an inefficient active muscle opening
  - prone to mechanical obstruction from enlarged adenoids
  - prone to functional obstruction, e.g., a floppy cartilaginous Eustachian tube

The Role of the Adenoids in the Pathogenesis of Acute Otitis Media

- Chronically-infected adenoids may provide a reservoir of pathogenic bacteria in the nasopharynx
- Enlarged adenoids may produce mechanical obstruction of the Eustachian tube
- Enlarged adenoids may produce functional obstruction of the Eustachian tube, with resultant, negative pressure in the middle ear.
- Enlarged adenoids may obstruct the posterior

choana, causing increased nasopharyngeal
pressure during swallowing, with insufflation
of bacteria into the middle ear via the
Eustachian tube

Microbiology of Acute Otitis Media

- The normal middle ear is sterile
- *Streptococcus pneumoniae* and *Haemophilus influenzae* are the two major pathogens in acute otitis media
- *Streptococcus pneumniae* is the most common cause of acute otitis media
- *Moraxella catarrhalis:* almost 80 percent of *M. catarrhalis* strains elaborate Beta-lactamase
- *Chlamydia trachomatis* is a rare cause of acute otitis media
- Bullous myringitis is not a distinct entity
- Mycoplasmas are no longer considered to be the causative organism in Bullous myringitis
- At present, Bullous myringitis is considered to be merely one manifestation of acute otitis media

The Primary Bacterial Pathogens in Acute, Suppurative Otitis Media

- There is an increasing frequency of resistant strains of pathogens in acute otitis media

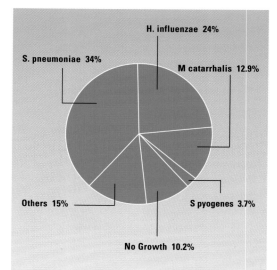

Chief bacterial pathogens isolated from middle-ear aspirates of infants and children with acute otitis media. *Source*: Bluestone CD: *Respiratory Infections Review* 1(1), 1993

- Beta-lactamase producing *Haemophilus influenzae*
- Beta-lactamase producing *Moraxella catarrhalis*

The Role of Beta-lactamase Producing Haemophilus influenzae in Acute Otitis Media

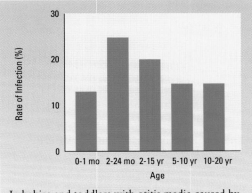

In babies and toddlers with otitis media caused by non-type b *H. influenzae*, up to 25% of infections were caused by beta-lactamase producing strains.
Source: Doern GV et al: *Antimicrobial Agents and Chemotherapy* 1988;32: 180-185

Otoscopic Appearances

- The otoscopic appearance of the tympanic membrane depends upon the stage of development and the severity of the infection
- While acute otitis media is usually a rapid and progressive infection, it has traditionally been divided into four stages, each with its own symptoms and otoscopic appearance:
  - the stage of Eustachian-tube obstruction
  - the stage of redness
  - the stage of suppuration
  - the stage of resolution

The Stage of Eustachian-tube Obstruction

- Minimal symptoms: slight discomfort or stuffiness in the ear
- The pars flaccida, upper fourth of the tympanic membrane, shows slight redness and swelling

The Stage of Redness

- There is increasing earache and stuffiness
- The constitutional symptoms of a systemic infection are usually present: fever, malaise, nausea and, in children, vomiting and/or diarrhea
- There is marked erythema of the tympanic membrane and vasodilatation of the radial vessels
- The vasodilatation may be so extensive that the entire surface of the eardrum becomes fiery red
- There is increased bulging of the pars flaccida
- A small amount of purulent exudate may be seen accumulating in the inferior portion of the tympanic cavity

The Stage of Suppuration

- This stage is characterized by severe local pain and an increase in the constitutional symptoms
- Most of the local pain appears to be caused by inflammation and stretching of the

tympanic membrane and its sensory nerves

- The purulent exudate collects under pressure within the middle ear, thereby forcing the tympanic membrane laterally (bulging)

- In severe cases, the bacteria and the infection spread into the tympanic membrane, causing edema of the eardrum and fluid seepage from its lateral surface

- This seepage may cause the keratin patches on the lateral surface of the tympanic membrane to swell

- In severe cases, the actual infection may spread through an area of the tympanic membrane and cause necrosis of the tiny vessels within the tympanic membrane

- These radial vessels may then rupture, producing areas of hemorrhage on the surface of the eardrum

- As the infection spreads through the tympanic membrane, it may also cause necrosis of the fibrous middle layer of the tympanic membrane. When this happens, the tympanic membrane loses its strength in this area. The result is usually a perforation of the tympanic membrane at this site of necrosis

- In this situation, the tympanic membrane can be considered the outer layer of an abscess cavity, which perforates to allow the pus that has accumulated within the middle ear to drain into the external auditory canal

- Such a perforation can be considered "nature's myringotomy"
- This is a much more desirable situation than having the abscess cavity rupture superiorly into the meningeal spaces

The Stage of Resolution

- The stage of resolution classically occurs after the tympanic membrane has perforated. The pain resolves dramatically, and the principal symptom is a transient, purulent otorrhea
- A small perforation, sometimes only the size of a pinhole, will be seen in the tympanic membrane, and purulent material will be seen in the external canal
- With the introduction of antibiotics, the traditional stage of resolution by perforation of the eardrum is less likely to occur. Instead, the suppurative process is often arrested, with either a gradual resolution of the infection, or the subsequent development of a mucoid effusion — mucoid otitis media

The Fluid

- Fluid within the middle ear is frankly purulent
- It is creamy white and contains large numbers of polymorphonuclear leukocytes and bacteria

Histopathology

- The mucosa of the middle-ear cleft shows the characteristic changes of acute inflammation: marked edema; vasodilatation, with a heavy infiltration by acute inflammatory cells and later by lymphocytes and plasma cells
- The tympanic membrane becomes edematous and hyperemic as the infection spreads into its layers
- The outer epithelial layer of the tympanic membrane proliferates with increased keratinocyte production and, ultimately, desquamation
- Localized necrosis of the fibrous middle layer of the tympanic membrane may occur, resulting in a perforation of the eardrum

Treatment

Principles of Therapy

- The mainstay of treatment is antibiotic therapy
- Choose a broad-spectrum antibiotic that is:
  - suitable for the most common pathogens
  - suitable for the treatment of Beta-lactamase producing bacteria
- Prescribe analgesics for pain
- A myringotomy may provide dramatic relief of pain

Acute Otitis Media: Therapeutic Principles

- Rational, antimicrobial therapy requires an understanding of the microbiologic cause of the infection. While, in an ideal situation, antimicrobial therapy should be based upon the result of a culture from the source of the infection, in otitis media, culture studies are usually impractical. Thus, empirical therapy must be instituted based upon the most likely probability that the infection is caused by the organisms.
- Antibiotics are the mainstay in the treatment of acute otitis media. The antibiotic chosen should have as complete a coverage as possible of the four primary pathogens in AOM:
  - *Streptococcus pneumoniae*
  - *Haemophilus influenzae*
  - *Moraxella catarrhalis*
  - *Streptococcus pyogenes*
- The antibiotic chosen should be as effective as possible against the two primary, resistant strains of pathogens in AOM:
  - Beta-lactamase producing *Haemophilus influenzae*
  - Beta-lactamase producing *Moraxella catarrhalis*

- The antibiotic should:
  - be proven effective
  - be safe
  - have a low incidence of side effects

Antibiotic Treatment of Acute Otitis Media

Newborns

- Suggest using the same initial therapy as recommended for older adults:
  - Amoxicillin with potassium clavulanate (PO 40 mg/kg/day divided into three doses Q 8 H), *or*
  - Cefaclor (PO 40 mg/kg/day divided into three doses Q 8 H)
  - May have an advantage, because of their increased activity, against coliforms and *Staphylococci,* which cause 10 to 20 percent of these cases.
- If there is no clinical improvement from therapy, a sample of the middle-ear fluid should be obtained for culture via tympanocentesis

Infants and Children

- Amoxicillin (40 mg/kg/day PO divided into three doses Q 8 H), *or*
- Amoxicillin with potassium clavulanate (40 mg/kg/day PO divided into three doses Q 8 H), *or*
- Cefaclor (40 mg/kg/day PO divided into three doses Q 8 H), *or*
- Erythromycin-sulfa combination (erythromycin component 40 mg/kg/day PO

divided into four doses Q 6 H), *or*
- Trimethoprim/sulfamethoxazole
  (6 to 8 mg/kg/day of the TMP component
  PO divided into two doses Q 12 hours, *or*
  Cefixime 8 mg/kg/day once daily *or* divided
  into two doses Q 12 hours)
- If the tympanic membrane has ruptured, then
  a sample of any discharge should be taken for
  Gram's stain and culture
- If there has been prior antibiotic therapy, or
  an immunocompromised host, one should
  suspect the presence of an unusual pathogen,
  and a sample of the middle-ear fluid should
  be obtained for culture by tympanocentesis

Persistent Otitis Media

- May be due to:
  - resistance of the bacteria to the antibiotic
    prescribed
  - an inadequate course of antibiotic (strength
    or duration)
- Consider a broad-spectrum antibiotic that is
  Beta-lactamase-resistant

Recurrent Otitis Media: a Special Problem

- May be due to:
  - an immunologic deficiency
  - an immunocompromised host
  - a new bacterial strain
  - enlarged or chronically-infected adenoids

Prevention of Recurrent Acute Otitis Media

- Antimicrobial chemoprophylaxis
- *Haemophilus influenza* type b vaccination
- Immunotherapy to reduce the effects of allergy
- Insertion of tympanostomy tubes to improve middle-ear ventilation
- Adenoidectomy, with or without tonsillectomy:
  - to improve Eustachian tube insufficiency, *and*
  - to remove a reservoir of nasopharyngeal pathogens

Reference

Nelson JD. 1991-1992 Pocketbook of Pediatric Antimicrobial Therapy, 9th ed. Williams & Wilkins, Baltimore MD, 1991.

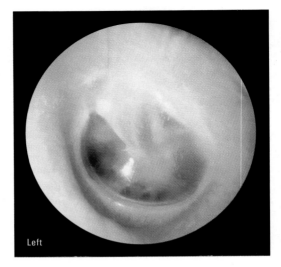

Left

Figure 1.1 Normal tympanic membrane

The normal tympanic membrane is a pale-grey, semitransparent membrane. The handle of the malleus can be seen in the middle of the tympanic membrane, running obliquely downwards and backwards. The long process of the incus can be seen through the posterior superior quadrant of the eardrum. Note the "cone of light" that extends antero-inferiorly from the lower end of the malleus, the umbo.

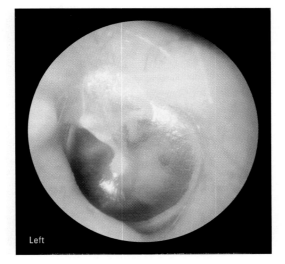

Left

Figure 1.2 Normal tympanic membrane

The inferior four fifths of the tympanic membrane have a distinct fibrous middle layer and are called the pars tensa. The upper fifth of the tympanic membrane has a sparse and flexible, fibrous middle layer. This tympanic membrane has a well-developed and prominent pars flaccida.

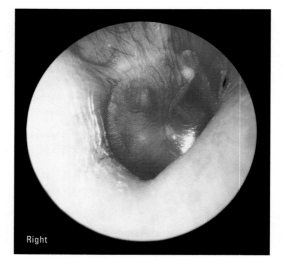

Right

Figure 1.3 Prominent vascular strip

The tiny vessels that run inferiorly along the handle of the malleus, the vascular strip, and the radial vessels that run across the surface of the tympanic membrane are not normally visible. This patient has a normally prominent vascular strip. This should not be confused with the early stages of an otitis media.

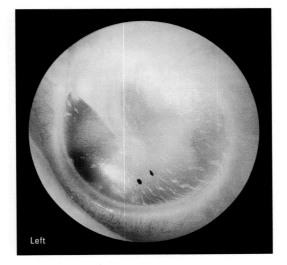

Left

Figure 1.4 Migrating ink dots

The surface of the tympanic membrane has a unique, self-cleansing action, which is the result of the epithelium's ability to migrate outwards in a centrifugal pattern. Note the two tiny dots of India ink that have been applied to this left tympanic membrane, in the six o'clock position.

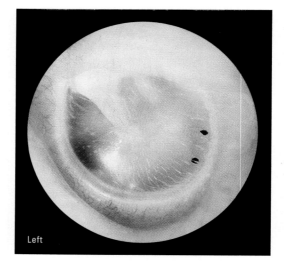

Left

Figure 1.5 Migrating ink dots
Two months later, the ink dots seen in the previous photograph have been carried laterally by the migratory action of the tympanic membrane and can now be seen adjacent to the annulus, in the three o'clock position.

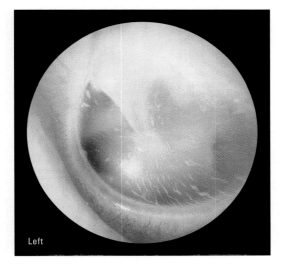

Left

Figure 1.6 Keratin patches

Small, radially-oriented, tiny, white patches or mounds of keratin squames can be seen, if the examiner looks carefully, on the surface of the normal tympanic membrane. These patches consist of older and thicker collections of keratin squames that have migrated centrifugally from the central portion of the tympanic membrane. The keratin patches are visible in the posterior inferior quadrant of this normal left tympanic membrane.

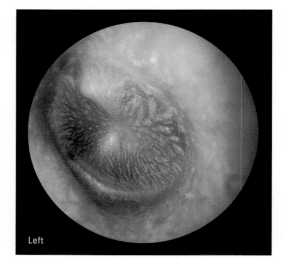

Left

Figure 1.7 Prominent keratin patches
Keratin patches are hydrophilic and swell
when exposed to water. Note the profusion of
prominent keratin patches on the surface of
this otherwise normal left tympanic membrane.

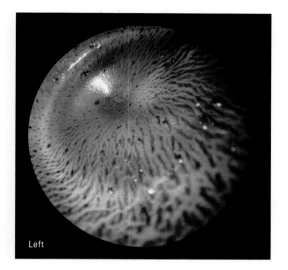

Left

Figure 1.8 Keratin patches stained with osmium

Keratin patches are always present, even when they cannot be seen. The shape and distribution of keratin patches can be seen clearly in this osmium-stained cadaveric specimen.

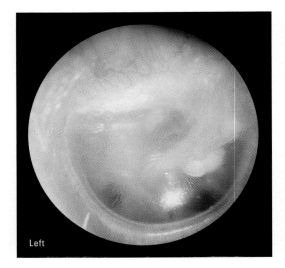

Left

Figure 1.9 Congenital cholesteatoma

The small, pearly-white mass protruding anteriorly from behind the anterior border of the
malleus is a congenital cholesteatoma arising
in the middle ear. These small, congenital,
epidermal, cyst-like structures can be removed
easily when they are small.

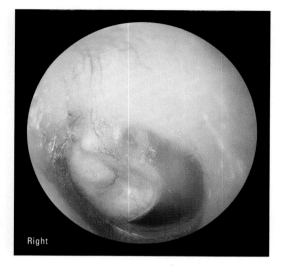

Right

Figure 1.10 Congenital cholesteatoma
The large, white mass seen behind the anterior inferior half of this tympanic membrane is a large, congenital cholesteatoma. The presence of any discrete white structure deep in the tympanic membrane should alert the examiner to the possibility of a congenital middle-ear cholesteatoma. Specialist referral is mandatory.

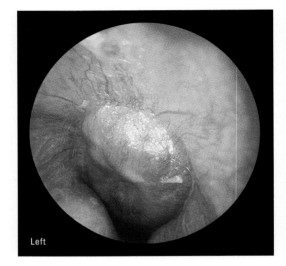

Left

Figure 1.11 Early, acute otitis media

The earliest visible otoscopic change in acute,
suppurative otitis media consists of redness,
edema and bulging of the pars flaccida. This
is the stage of Eustachian-tube obstruction.

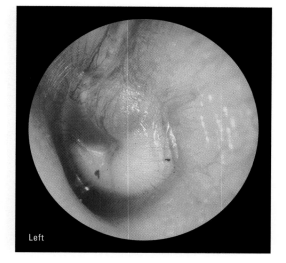

Left

Figure 1.12 Early acute otitis media

Shortly after, a creamy-white, purulent effusion can be seen collecting in the middle ear. This is the stage of redness.

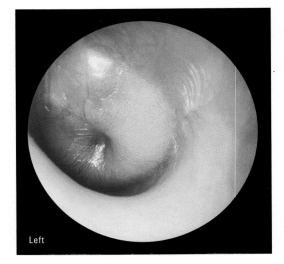

Left

Figure 1.13 Acute otitis media

The middle ear then becomes completely filled with the purulent exudate, the pressure of which causes the tympanic membrane to bulge laterally. This is the stage of suppuration.

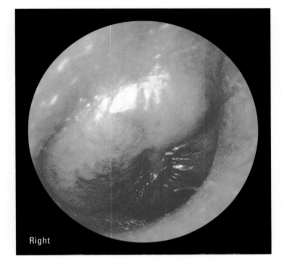

Right

Figure 1.14 Severe, acute otitis media
The infection in the middle ear may extend
into the tympanic membrane, causing infection and necrosis with rupture of the radial
vessels. Note the central area of interstitial
hemorrhage.

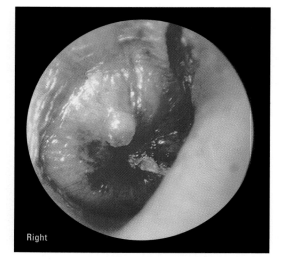

Right

Figure 1.15 Severe acute otitis media
The infection in the middle ear may spread
into the fibrous middle layer of the tympanic
membrane, causing necrosis of a portion of
the fibrous middle layer. The small herniation
seen in the center of this right tympanic membrane, just posterior to the mid-portion of the
malleus, represents such a necrotic area. The
tympanic membrane has lost its strength in
the area of necrosis, and the pressure of the
purulent effusion within the middle ear has
caused the epithelium to bulge laterally. This
is the area through which a perforation will
shortly develop.

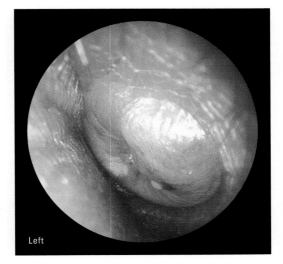

Left

Figure 1.16 Acute otitis media

This patient presented with an acute otitis
media in the stage of suppuration. Note the
redness and bulging of the pars flaccida and
the accumulation of a creamy-white, purulent
exudate in the middle ear. There is a moderate outward bulging of the eardrum.

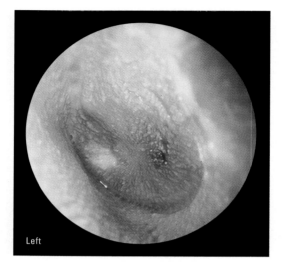

Left

Figure 1.17 Acute otitis media

This is the same patient 24 hours later, in the
stage of resolution. The purulent exudate in
the middle ear has drained into the external
auditory canal through a tiny, pin-hole perforation that developed through the tiny area of
herniation, which can be seen in the previous
photograph just anterior to the inferior portion of the malleus.

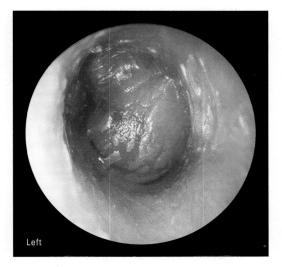

Left

Figure 1.18 Severe, acute otitis media

In some severe cases, the tympanic membrane may bulge outwards to such an extent that all the normal landmarks are obscured.

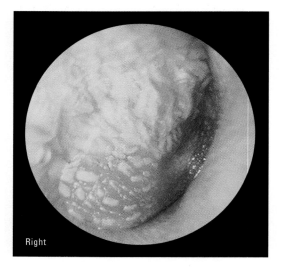

Right

Figure 1.19 Severe, acute otitis media
In this patient, the infection in the middle ear
has extended through the bulging tympanic
membrane. Note the swollen keratin patches
on the lateral surface of the tympanic membrane.

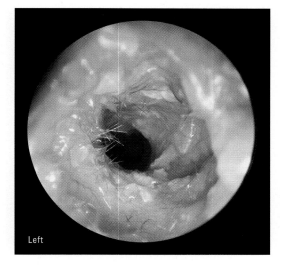

Left

Figure 1.20 The stage of resolution
With the release of purulent material into the
external auditory canal, the tympanic membrane has ruptured. This is the stage of resolution.

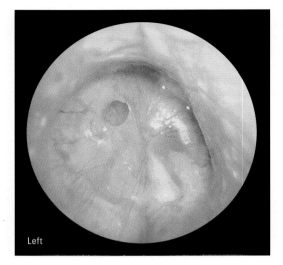

Left

Figure 1.21 The stage of resolution
The small, central perforation in this left tympanic membrane is the result of an episode of acute otitis media three weeks previously. This perforation can be considered to be "nature's myringotomy."

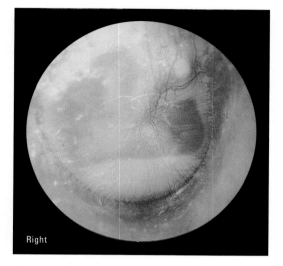

Right

Figure 1.22 The stage of resolution

The stage of resolution may be modified
through antibiotic therapy. This patient had
an acute otitis media two weeks previously.
Note the air fluid level and the collection of
white and presumably sterile exudate in the
inferior third of the middle ear.

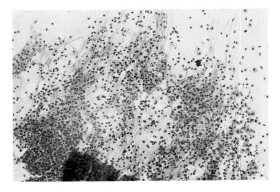

Figure 1.23 The purulent effusion

This is an H&E-stained smear of the pus, aspirated by tympanocentesis from the middle ear of a patient with acute, suppurative otitis media. Note the numerous, acute, inflammatory cells.

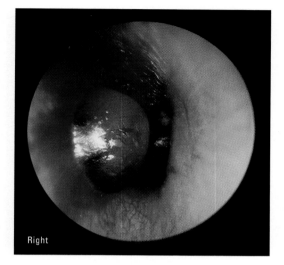

Right

Figure 1.24 Bullous myringitis

Bullous myringitis is a distinctive form of
acute otitis media that is characterized by
severe local pain, and by the appearance of
hemorrhagic and serum-filled blisters on the
tympanic membrane and on the skin of the
adjacent, external auditory canal. The large
serum bulla seen on the posterior canal wall
contains a small collection of blood in the
dependent portion.

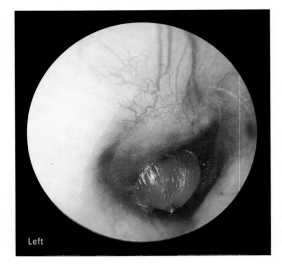

Figure 1.25 Bullous myringitis
A large, serum-filled bulla can be seen on the central portion of this left tympanic membrane.

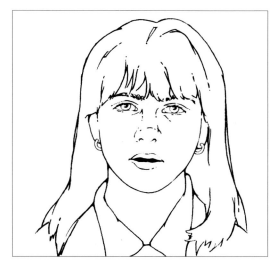

Figure 1.26 Adenoid facies

Hypertrophy of the nasopharyngeal pad of lymphoid tissue, the adenoids, is the most common cause of nasal obstruction in children. The most common presenting symptoms are chronic mouth breathing and snoring. The most dangerous symptom is sleep apnea. Adenoid hypertrophy is associated with an increased incidence of both acute otitis media and mucoid otitis media. Persistent mouth breathing due to nasal obstruction in childhood may result in the "long-face syndrome," previously called "adenoid facies."

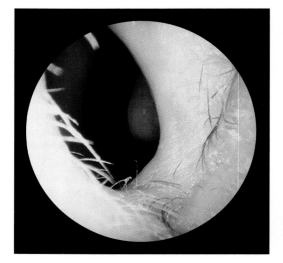

Figure 1.27 Anterior nasal, mucosal changes secondary to chronic nasopharyngeal obstruction from enlarged adenoid: "the small purple turbinate syndrome." When the air flow through the nasal cavity ceases as a result of enlarged adenoids, characteristic, secondary changes in the mucosa of the anterior nasal cavity may be observed. These changes consist of a state of vasoconstriction and purple discoloration of the mucosa of the anterior portion of the inferior turbinates. They result in a wider-than-normal anterior air space and pale-purple, small inferior turbinates. Such changes should not be misinterpreted as an allergic rhinitis.

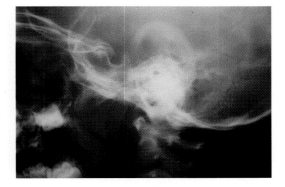

Figure 1.28 Adenoid hypertrophy (lateral radiograph)

Enlarged adenoids are not easily identified on physical examination. A lateral radiograph of the nasopharynx provides a simple and cost-effective method of assessing the size of the adenoids and the amount of post-nasal air space remaining.

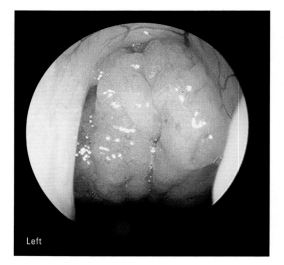

Left

Figure 1.29 Adenoid hypertrophy: endoscopic view

Enlarged adenoids extending anteriorly into and obstructing the left posterior choana are clearly seen in this endoscopic photograph. While the adenoid tonsil usually undergoes spontaneous involution around puberty, the hypertrophy may persist into adult life. Adenoid hypertrophy in adults may be associated with an HIV positivity.

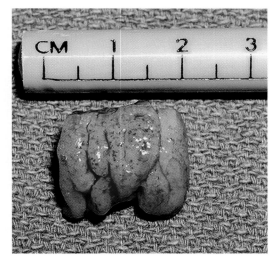

Figure 1.30 Adenoids (surgical specimen)

When obstruction of the nasopharynx causes total nasal obstruction, snoring, recurrent otitis media, secondary dental problems, or sleep apnea, then adenoidectomy is indicated. Surgical removal of the adenoids is a relatively safe and painless procedure. This huge adenoid tonsil was removed from the nasopharynx of a six-year-old child.

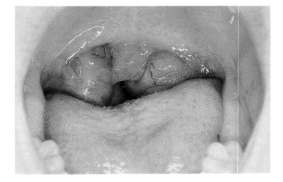

Figure 1.31 Tonsillar hypertrophy
There is no convincing correlation between
tonsillar hypertrophy and otitis media. For
this reason, tonsillectomy is currently only
considered as an adjunct to adenoidectomy in
the rare problem case.

2

CASTS AND CRUSTS OF THE TYMPANIC MEMBRANE

Definition

- A tympanic membrane crust is a collection of keratinocytes and inspissated serum that are attached to the lateral surface of the tympanic membrane
- A cast is a crust that has spontaneously separated from the surface of the eardrum

Etiology

Casts

- Over time, once the inflammation within the middle ear and tympanic membrane has resolved, the normal process of epithelial migration on the surface of the tympanic membrane will separate the crust from the lateral surface of the tympanic membrane, at which point the "crust" becomes known as a "cast"
- The medial surface of a cast usually duplicates the contours of the lateral surface of the underlying tympanic membrane

Crusts

- In severe cases of acute otitis media, crust formation on the lateral surface of the tympanic membrane is the result of the local infection's or inflammation's spread from the middle ear into the tympanic membrane
- The tympanic-membrane inflammation stimulates the outer epithelial layer of the eardrum, thereby causing a proliferation of the outer surface layer of keratinocytes
- Due to a local inhibition of the enzymes that are responsible for the normal separation and migration of the surface layer of keratinocytes, stratified keratinocytes accumulate rapidly on the surface of the tympanic membrane
- The serous fluid, which is exuded by the inflamed eardrum, is imbibed by this layer of hydrophilic keratinocytes, which then swell
- This rapidly-accumulating mixture of inflammatory exudate and keratinocytes outstrips the reserves of the normally efficient epithelial migration and cleaning, and a crust is formed on the lateral surface of the tympanic membrane

Otoscopic Appearance

- Tympanic-membrane crusts and casts are golden-yellow in color, semitranslucent and have a cracked or brittle consistency

Histopathology

- Both crusts and casts consist of multiple layers of adherent keratinocytes, embedded in an amorphous, eosinophilic exudate
- Degenerating leukocytes and entrapped bacteria are often seen scattered throughout the exudate

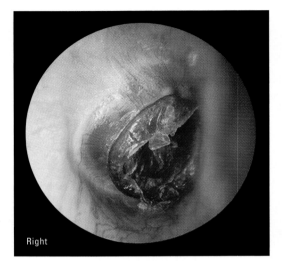

Right

Figure 2.1 Crust on tympanic membrane

A large crust has formed on the surface of this
left tympanic membrane during a previous,
severe bout of acute, suppurative otitis media.
The crust has already separated from the posterior portion of the now normal tympanic
membrane. Given time, tympanic membrane
crusts will separate spontaneously from the
tympanic membrane.

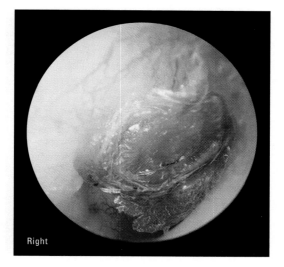

Right

Figure 2.2 Cast of tympanic membrane
Once a crust has completely separated from
the surface of the tympanic membrane, it is
called a "cast." Note the typical yellow, brittle, semitransparent consistency of the cast.

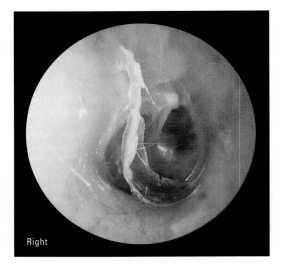

Right

Figure 2.3 Partial cast of tympanic membrane

A partial cast can be seen, which has recently separated from the posterior surface of this now normal tympanic membrane. Over time, tympanic membrane casts are carried out of the external auditory canal by the normal migratory action of the underlying epithelium.

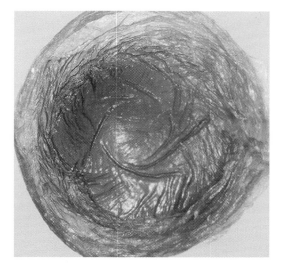

Figure 2.4 Total cast of tympanic membrane
The lateral surface of a complete cast of the
tympanic membrane. Note the yellow,
translucent nature of the cast.

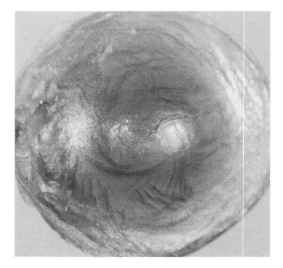

Figure 2.5 Total cast of tympanic membrane
The medial surface of the same cast. Note
how the medial surface of the cast mirrors the
lateral surface of the tympanic membrane
from which it has separated.

MASTOIDITIS

Definition

• Acute mastoiditis is an acute infection of
the air cells and of the bony walls (septa) of
the mastoid air cell system. These bony septa
eventually break down (coalesce) with the
accumulation of pus within the mastoid
process. Mastoiditis is a potentially life-
threatening disease, as the infection within the
mastoid can spread outside its confines to
enter the cranial cavity and cause meningitis
and or brain abscess.

Etiology

• Acute mastoiditis is a relatively infrequent
sequela of inadequately or incompletely treated
acute suppurative otitis media. Inadequate
treatment allows the infection to smolder in a
relatively asymptomatic manner, and to extend
beyond the mucosal lining of the   middle-ear
cleft into the adjacent bone. The result is an
osteitis and coalescence of the mastoid process.
• In order to avoid the development of mastoiditis, all cases of acute, suppurative otitis
media should be closely followed until a complete resolution has been obtained.

Symptoms

- Unfortunately, the symptoms of mastoiditis may be minimal and nonspecific, until the pus within the mastoid process is released. Hopefully this occurs into the external auditory canal or through the periosteum on the lateral surface of the mastoid, resulting in subperiosteal abscess, and not superiorly through the roof of the mastoid, i.e., into the middle cranial fossa as meningitis or brain abscess.
- Lassitude
- Low-grade fever
- Elevated white-blood count (WBC)
- Minimal discomfort or pressure in the affected ear

Otoscopic Appearance

- There are no pathognomonic otoscopic features. The tympanic membrane usually has those features that suggest a chronic or persistent acute suppurative process, showing a creamy white purulent exudate under pressure. This causes the drum to bulge outwards, and vasodilatation of the vessels over the surface of the drum is frequently present. The examiner may well be unable to determine if he/she is looking at a case of resolving acute, suppurative otitis media or chronic, acute, suppurative otitis media.

Diagnostic Tests

- The most important diagnostic test is the CT scan

Treatment

- Any patient suspected of developing acute mastoiditis should immediately be referred to a specialist, as an emergency mastoidectomy may be required

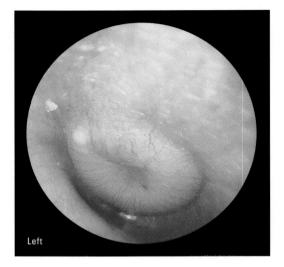

Left

Figure 3.1 Mastoiditis

In some cases of incompletely-treated, acute, suppurative otitis media, the infection within the middle-ear cleft may persist in a chronic and indolent form, and spread throughout the mastoid air cell system and into the bony septa that separate these mastoid cells. There are no pathognomonic, otoscopic features. The middle ear is filled with a creamy-white, purulent exudate under pressure, which causes the drum to bulge outwards. Note the vasodilatation of the vessels over the surface of the drum.

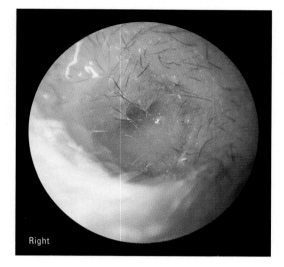

Right

Figure 3.2 Mastoiditis
The infection within the mastoid bone has ruptured through the posterior bony canal wall. The deep canal is filled with a creamy-white, purulent discharge.

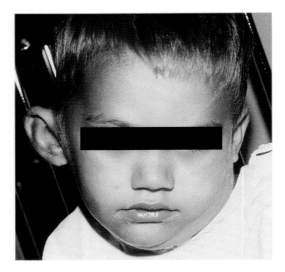

Figure 3.3 Mastoiditis with subperiosteal abscess formation

The infection in the mastoid has perforated the lateral surface of the mastoid cortex and produced a subperiosteal abscess. Note the characteristic displacement of the pinna in a lateral and downwards direction.

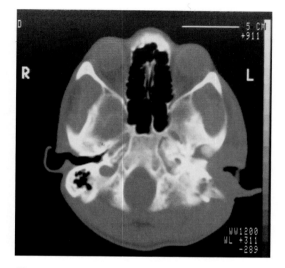

Figure 3.4 Acute mastoiditis with subperiosteal abscess CT scan

There is marked demineralization and coalescence of the bone of the left mastoid process. The obtuse angle of the postauricular sulcus and the swelling of the soft tissues of the posterior, external auditory canal are the result of the subperiosteal abscess.

4

....

MUCOID OTITIS MEDIA

Synonyms

- Otitis media with effusion (OME)
- Secretory otitis media
- Middle-ear catarrh
- "Glue ear"
- Catarrhal otitis media
- Tubotympanitis

Definition

- Mucoid otitis media is a chronic inflammation or infection of the mucosal lining of the middle-ear cleft, a chronic form of otitis media that is characterized by the accumulation of a thick, opalescent, mucoid, nonpurulent effusion within the middle-ear cleft.

Epidemiology

- Primarily a disease of children
- Most common cause of conductive hearing loss in children
- Can be diagnosed otoscopically

Predisposing Factors for Mucoid Otitis Media (MOM)

Sex

- More common in males

Age

- More common between two and six years of age
- Rare after the age of nine, the age by which the immune system has usually matured

Seasonal Variation

- More common during the winter months, December through March

Breast Feeding

- Decreased incidence in children who are breast-fed for at least three months

Nasal Obstruction

- More common in children with a history of nasal obstruction
- More common in children with mouth breathing
- More common in children who snore
- More common in children with enlarged adenoids

Previous Episodes of Acute Otitis Media

- More common in children with a previous episode of AOM
- Even more common in children with three or more annual episodes of AOM
- More common in children with a recent (one month or less) episode of AOM

Environmental

- More common in children of mothers who are heavy smokers, i.e., 15 or more cigarettes per day

Socioeconomic

- More common in children of the lower socioeconomic classes

Eustachian-tube Dysfunction

- Increased incidence in children with unrepaired cleft-palate deformity or other craniofacial abnormalities, which cause functional Eustachian-tube insufficiency
- Increased incidence in children with high, arched palates
- Increased incidence in children with Down's syndrome

Microbiology of Mucoid Otitis Media

- *Haemophilus influenzae* is the most common bacterial pathogen isolated from cases of mucoid otitis media.
- 95 percent of the *Haemophilus influenzae* isolates are unencapsulated and thus not typable with the antisera specific for the six recognized capsular types. At present, biotyping is the only available framework for the classification of this group of antigenically diverse organisms.

- The majority of the strains of *Haemophilus influenzae* isolated from patients with mucoid otitis media belonged to biotypes II and III. The incidence of Beta-lactamase production was 17 percent.

The Role of Bacterial Endotoxin in Middle-Ear Effusions

- *Haemophilus influenzae* have a lipopolysaccharide endotoxin attached to their surface
- Bacterial endotoxin is an extremely biologically-active material, a potent indicia of inflammation and a modulator of the immune response
- The bacterial endotoxin may be responsible for the persistence of a middle-ear effusion, long after the gram negative bacteria trapped within the middle ear are no longer viable
- Bacterial endotoxin is present in a high percentage of middle-ear effusions

Polymorphonuclear Leukocytes and Mucoid Effusions

- A strong association exists between an increased number of Polymorphonuclear leukocytes in the middle-ear effusion and the presence of *Streptococcus pneumoniae* and *Haemophilus influenzae*
- Through the release of lysosomal hydrolases, the Polymorphonuclear leukocytes contribute

to chronic middle-ear inflammation
* The eradication of these bacteria from the middle-ear space of children with mucoid otitis media may help to resolve the disease process by disrupting the host responses that maintain local inflammation, as well as the resulting effusion

The Role of Beta-Lactamase Producing Haemophilus Influenzae in Mucoid Otitis Media

Pathogen	Incidence		% producing beta-lactamase	
	1980	1989	1981	1989
S. pneumoniae	28%	44%	–	–
H. influenzae	20%	22%	21%	40%
M. (B) catarrhalis	9%	14%	68%	90%

The prevalence of *S. pneumoniae, H, influenzae and M. (B.) catarrhalis* is rising, and they are producing beta-lactamase more often. *Source*: Bluestone CD et al: *Journal of Pediatric Infectious Disease* 1992;11: S7-S11

Pathophysiology of Mucoid Otitis Media

- The normal response of the middle-ear mucosa to inflammation is the primary cause of mucoid otitis media

- The ascent of a viral upper-respiratory infection into the middle ear, via the Eustachian tube, appears to be the most frequent cause of this middle-ear inflammation

- A previous and incompletely resolved episode of acute otitis media is another common cause of middle-ear inflammation

- The delicate balance of the normal mucociliary transportation mechanism is abruptly upset in mucoid otitis media

- Responding to the inflammation, the middle-ear mucosa attempts to rid itself of the inciting cause by developing an increased number of mucous glands, and by increasing both the amount and the viscosity of the mucous produced

- The result is a middle-ear cleft that is filled with a thick, opalescent, mucoid, nonpurulent effusion

- The incidence of mucoid otitis media has increased greatly since the onset of the antibiotic era

- The use of antibiotics arrests the acute infectious process and prevents the "normal," full-fledged suppurative process with the forma-

tion of nature's "spontaneous myringotomy."
That is, a perforation forms instead and
allows the development of low-grade forms of
infection and chronic inflammation, such as is
seen within the middle-ear mucosa in MOM

Symptoms

- Mucoid otitis media is primarily a disease of
  young children; consequently, it is a relatively silent disease, in which the symptoms
  are minimal, vague and, unfortunately, easily
  overlooked
- The most important symptom is conductive
  hearing loss, which is present when the disease affects both ears
- This conductive loss may be quite significant,
  i.e., up to 45 to 50 decibels
- The effects of the hearing loss may only
  appear in relatively subtle forms of inatten-
  tion, slow speech and language development,
  irritability and poor performance at school

Otoscopic Appearance

- The otoscopic picture in mucoid otitis media
  is more varied than seen in serous otitis media
- The otoscopic picture depends upon the
  amount of inflammation present in the middle
  ear and the amount and character of the effusion within the middle ear
- The presence of the thick, opalescent mucoid
  exudate within the middle ear is responsible

for the dull texture and the pearly-grey color
of the tympanic membrane
- Because the exudate within the middle ear is
opalescent, one cannot see into the depths
of the middle ear (in contrast to serous otitis
media); the eardrum loses its semitrans-
parency
- Air fluid levels are uncommon (in contrast to
serous otitis media).
- The radial vessels of the tympanic membrane
are frequently dilated, especially when there
has been a prior episode of acute otitis media
(in contrast to serous otitis media)
- The tympanic membrane is usually not
retracted and may instead be flattened, or
there may even be an outward bulging of the
eardrum (in contrast to serous otitis media)

The Fluid

- In serous otitis media, is a true exudate
- Opalescent, pearly-grey in color, extremely
thick and tenacious in consistency
- Viscosity of the effusion is due to the presence
of rheologically-active mucous glycoproteins,
mucins
- Histologically, the effusion stains a dark pink
to light purple with H&E
- Many chronic inflammatory cells within the
fluid

Histopathology

- Mucosa of the middle ear undergoes numerous changes in MOM
- Mucosa is grossly thickened and edematous
- Surface of the mucosa becomes covered with a tall, ciliated epithelium
- Number of goblet cells increases
- Marked vasodilatation of the submucosal vessels
- Increase in both the number and size of mucous glands in the subepithelial layers
- Subepithelial layer swells up to four or five times its normal thickness
- Large numbers of subepithelial mucous cysts, filled with inspissated mucous, appear in the subepithelial layer

Treatment

The key elements of treatment include:

- administration of a suitable broad-spectrum antibiotic to sterilize the middle-ear effusion
  - suitable for the most common pathogens
  - suitable for the treatment of Beta-lactamase, producing bacteria
- observation alone: 90 percent of middle-ear effusions will clear spontaneously within three months
- judicious use of myringotomy and myringotomy with ventilation-tube insertion
- judicious use of adenoidectomy, with or without tonsillectomy in problem cases

Mucoid Otitis Media: Therapeutic Principles

• An appropriate antibiotic should be used to sterilize the effusion within the middle ear

• The thick, mucoid effusion within the middle ear can be expected to persist for several weeks prior to clearing

• Given sufficient time, up to three months, the majority of middle-ear effusions will resolve spontaneously

Persistance of Middle-ear Effusion

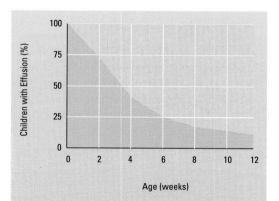

Middle-ear effusion persists for weeks to months after an episode of acute otitis media. Appropriate antimicrobial agents sterilize the middle ear effusion but do not clear the the fluid from the middle-ear space. *Source*: Klein JO: Pediatrics 71(4) 640, 1983

The Potential Sequelae of Persistent Mucoid Otitis Media

- These children have a predisposition to recurring bouts of otitis media
- Many children are functionally deaf while the mucoid effusion remains in the middle ear
- The hearing loss may be as great as 45 decibels
- This persistent hearing loss may lead to:
  - delayed speech and language development
  - learning impairment, as demonstrated by lower scores on tests of vocabulary, auditory comprehension and verbal ability
  - attention deficits
- Chronic intratympanic negative pressure, and/or recurrent episodes of middle-ear infection, may cause irreversible middle-ear damage, e.g., tympanosclerosis, retraction pockets, ossicular erosion, perforation and cholesteatoma

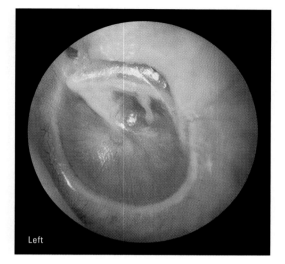

Left

Figure 4.1 Mucoid otitis media

The otoscopic appearance of mucoid otitis media is quite variable and depends upon the degree of inflammation present and the amount of exudate remaining in the middle ear. At first glance, this left tympanic membrane appears to be normal; however, on careful inspection it is apparent that the middle ear is filled with a grey fluid. Note how opalescence of the fluid prevents the examiner from seeing "into" the middle ear.

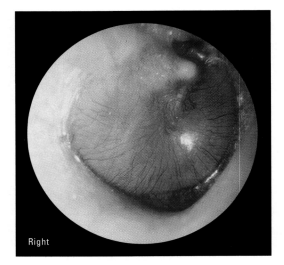

Right

Figure 4.2 Mucoid otitis media
The creamy-white fluid in this right middle
ear has given the tympanic membrane a
whitish discoloration. Note the prominent
dilatation of the radial vessels. This combination of a white coloration and vasodilatation
suggests the presence of continuing, low-grade
infection. The use of a suitable antibiotic is
advisable in such a case.

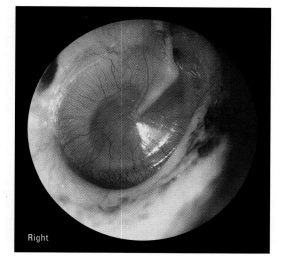

Right

Figure 4.3 Mucoid otitis media
The tympanic membrane shows a similar
appearance to that seen in the previous photograph. Note the retraction of the central portion of the tympanic membrane.

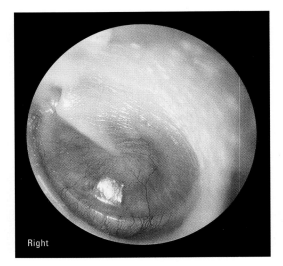

Right

Figure 4.4 Mucoid otitis media

This is the opposite ear of the patient shown in the previous photograph. The middle ear is filled with a typical, opalescent, glue-like fluid that prevents the examiner from viewing the medial wall of the middle ear.

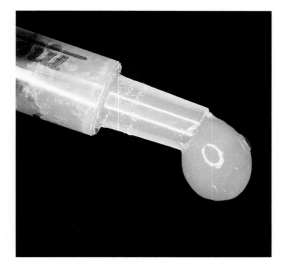

Figure 4.5 Mucoid fluid
The typical appearance of the fluid removed
from the middle ears of children with mucoid
otitis media. The effusion is thick, opalescent,
viscid, and has a creamy-yellow coloration.
The usual volume of fluid aspirated is
between 0.1 to 0.2 ml.

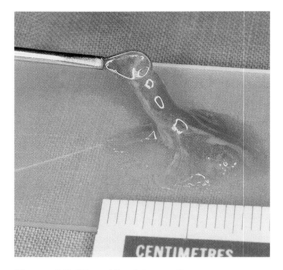

Figure 4.6 Mucoid otitis media

The tenacious and glue-like nature of the mucoid effusion is shown.

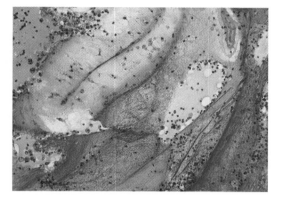

Figure 4.7 Histology of the mucoid effusion
Histologically, the effusion stains a dark
pink to light purple color with hematoxylin
and eosin. The strands of thick mucous
give the mucoid effusion an irregular, stain-
ing appearance. Note the large numbers of
chronic, inflammatory cells present within the
effusion.

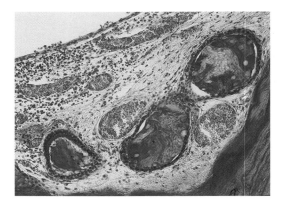

Figure 4.8 Histology of the mucoid otitis media

The mucosa of the middle ear undergoes numerous changes in mucoid otitis media: the mucosa is grossly thickened and edematous, there is marked vasodilatation of the submucosal vessels, and there is an increase in both the number and size of the mucous glands in the subepithelial layers. Note the dense infiltration by chronic inflammatory cells of the subepithelial layer.

5

SEROUS OTITIS MEDIA

Definition

- Not a true "otitis" media, as there is no infection or inflammation
- Characterized by the accumulation of a clear, thin, golden-yellow, serous transudate in the middle-ear cleft

Epidemiology

- Primarily a disease of adults
- After wax impaction, the most common cause of conductive hearing loss in adults
- Can be diagnosed otoscopically
- In persistent or recurrent cases of serous otitis media, one must rule out carcinoma of the nasopharynx

Pathophysiology of Serous Otitis Media

- The middle-ear cleft is a noncollapsable, gas-filled body cavity that communicates intermittently with the outside atmosphere via the Eustachian tube
- The Eustachian tube is normally closed
- The Eustachian tube opens several times a minute for brief intervals, during swallowing or yawning

- These brief openings allow the equalization of the middle-ear pressure with the ambient, atmospheric air pressure
- These brief openings also permit a partial exchange of the gaseous contents of the middle-ear cavity
- Normal middle-ear gas composition:
  - nitrogen 88 percent
  - oxygen 10 percent
  - carbon dioxide 2 percent
- Serous otitis media is the result of Eustachian-tube obstruction, which causes a chain of events that has been termed "hydrops ex vacuo," water out of a vacuum

Hydrops ex vacuo

- This deprivation of the middle-ear's air supply prevents replacement of the air within the middle ear
- The air within the middle ear is gradually absorbed by the mucosa lining of the middle-ear cleft
- This produces a partial vacuum, negative pressure within the middle ear
- Over time, this negative, intratympanic pressure gradually draws a serous transudate from the capillaries of the mucosa of the middle ear
- The result is a gradual filling of the middle-ear cleft with a golden-yellow, clear fluid

Causes of Eustachian-tube Obstruction

- Viral upper-respiratory tract infection is the most common cause
- Respiratory-tract allergy
- Enlarged adenoids
- Otitic barotrauma
- Tumors of the nasopharynx, especially carcinoma of the nasopharynx
- Cleft-palate deformity

Symptoms

- Hearing loss
- A blocked or stuffy feeling in the ear
- Popping on swallowing
- Unlike children with mucoid otitis media, adults are quite aware of their symptoms and will readily seek medical attention

Otoscopic Features

- Golden-yellow to orange-colored clear transudate within the middle ear colors the tympanic membrane
- As there is neither infection nor inflammation present, the tympanic membrane appears otherwise normal
- Because the transudate is clear, one can see "through" the fluid into the depths, to the medial wall of the middle ear
- When there is a high level of negative intratympanic pressure, the tympanic membrane

will be "sucked" medially, i.e., retracted
- Retraction of the tympanic membrane causes the handle of the malleus to appear foreshortened and the lateral process of the malleus to appear unusually prominent

Further Investigations

- Tympanometry is useful in identifying the patient with abnormal middle-ear pressures or decreased tympanic-membrane mobility
- Audiometry is useful in identifying and quantifying the hearing loss

The Fluid

- A true transudate
- Clear, watery, golden-yellow to orange in color
- No cells within the fluid

Histopathology

- No histopathologic evidence of infection or inflammation
- No histopathologic changes within the middle-ear cleft
- Mucoperiosteum lining the middle-ear cleft is thin and normal in appearance
- Histologically, the serous transudate appears as a homogenous eosinophilic acellular transudate when stained with H&E

Treatment

- Treatment is aimed at re-aeration of the middle ear, either through:
  - restoration of eustachian-tube function, performing Valsalva's maneuver: inhaling, closing the mouth, pinching the nostril closed and then attempting to exhale forcefully through the nose against the closed nostrils (autoinflation)
  - bypassing the Eustachian tube by inserting a ventilation tube through the tympanic membrane, *or*
  - observation alone
- Systemic and topical decongestants are of dubious value

Table 5.1   Distinguishing Characteristics of Mucoid Otitis Media and Serous Otitis Media

Characteristic	Mucoid otitis media	Serous otitis media
Type of fluid	Inflammatory exudate	Passive transudate
Etiology	Inflammation or infection of the mucosal lining of middle ear cleft	Eustachian tube obstruction producing hydrops ex vacuo
Fluid consistency	Thick	Thin
Fluid cell content	Many inflammatory cells	No cells
Hearing loss	30 to 40 dB	20 to 30 dB
Histopathologic changes in the middle ear mucosa	Edema, hyperemia, mucous, gland hypertrophy, chronic inflammatory cell infiltration	None

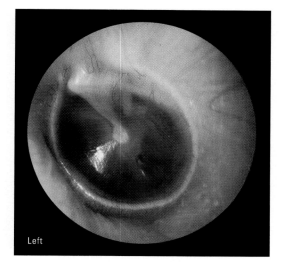

Left

Figure 5.1 Serous otitis media

Serous otitis media is characterized by the presence of a thin, straw-colored, clear transudate in the middle ear. The tympanic membrane shows an orange discoloration from the fluid that fills the middle-ear cleft. The clear nature of the fluid allows the examiner to look into the depths of the middle ear.

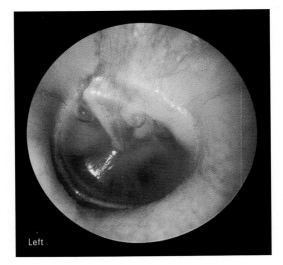

Left

Figure 5.2 Serous otitis media prior to autoinflation

This adult patient developed a serous otitis media following an upper-respiratory infection.

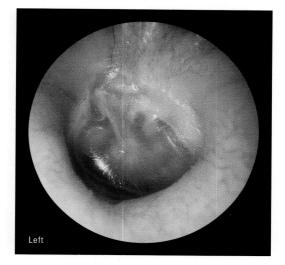

Left

Figure 5.3 Serous otitis media post autoinflation

This is the same patient seen in the previous photograph, approximately ten minutes later. The patient has performed a Valsalva maneuver, autoinflation, which forced air up the Eustachian tube into the middle ear and displaced the serous transudate out of the middle ear.

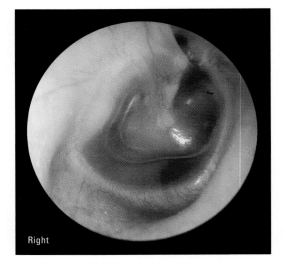

Right

Figure 5.4 Serous otitis media air-fluid level
This patient has an air-fluid level following
autoinflation. Note the orange color of the
transudate.

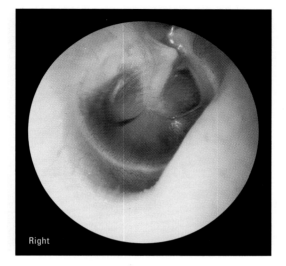

Right

Figure 5.5 Resolving serous otitis media with air-fluid levels

The serous otitis media in this patient is resolving spontaneously. Note the crescent-shaped menisci anterior and posterior to the lower portion of the malleus.

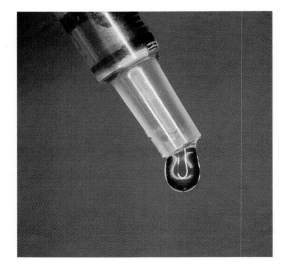

Figure 5.6 Serous otitis media: the transudate

The fluid within the middle ear in serous otitis media is a thin, clear, golden-yellow, watery transudate.

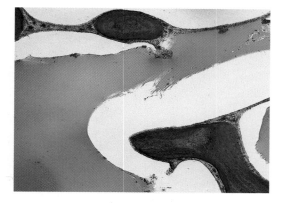

Figure 5.7 Histology of the transudate
Histologically, the serous transudate appears
as a homogenous eosinophilic acellular transudate when stained with H&E.

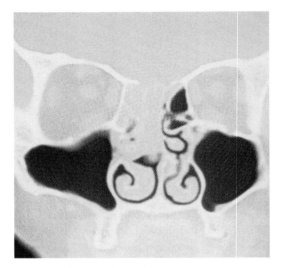

Figure 5.8 Nasopharyngeal carcinoma causing serous otitis media

Carcinoma of the nasopharynx is the most common malignancy of the nasopharynx. It is asymptomatic in its early stages and may only present as eustachian-tube obstruction with persistent or recurrent serous otitis media. While nasopharyngeal carcinoma occurs more commonly in orientals, no racial group is immune to this insidious tumor.

6

INDICATIONS FOR TYMPANOCENTESIS OR MYRINGOTOMY

- Otitis media in a seriously-ill or toxic patient
- Suppurative complications
- For the relief of severe pain
- When there has been an unsatisfactory response to antibiotic therapy, both for treatment and diagnosis
- For microbiologic diagnosis in those situations where the presence of an unusual pathogen is suspected, e.g., in newborns and in immunodeficient hosts

Tympanocentesis, Myringotomy, and Ventilation Tubes

Tympanocentesis: trans-tympanic needle aspiration of the middle ear. Tympanocentesis is performed to obtain a sample of middle-ear fluid for microbiologic study

Myringotomy: an incision through the tympanic membrane. A myringotomy is usually performed to allow access to the middle ear in order to aspirate the middle-ear contents for either diagnostic or therapeutic purposes

Tympanostomy: the insertion of a ventilation tube through the tympanic membrane. Most myringotomy incisions heal within one week and, if the Eustachian tube and the middle-ear mucosa have not returned to normal after the procedure, the effusion within the middle ear will recur

Tympanostomy-tube Design Features

- All tubes have a central lumen that allows the passage of gases and secretions
- All tubes have an inner flange that prevents the tube from falling out of the drum prematurely
- All tubes have either a long shaft or an outer flange that prevents the tube from falling medially into the middle ear

Functions of a Tympanostomy Tube

- Ventilation tubes serve three prime functions:
  - aeration of the middle ear
  - equalization of the pressure within the middle ear to that of the surrounding atmosphere ; *and*
  - the provision of a drainage pathway from the middle ear, should an otitis media develop
- This is why these tubes have been referred to by a number of different names: ventilation tubes, pressure-equalization tubes, drain tubes, artificial Eustachian tubes, and tympanostomy tubes.

Indications for the Use of Tympanostomy Tubes

- For treatment of persistent, more than three months' duration, mucoid otitis media that has not responded to appropriate medical therapy
- For the prevention of recurrent episodes of acute otitis media, e.g., four or more episodes over 12 months
- For the prevention of recurrent episodes of mucoid otitis media, e.g., four or more episodes over 12 months
- For the treatment of the hearing loss caused by mucoid effusion, when the hearing loss is causing learning or social difficulties
- For the treatment of Eustachian-tube dysfunction
- For the treatment of those middle-ear problems caused by chronic eustachian-tube dysfunction, e.g., retraction pockets, ossicular erosion, atelectasis of the middle ear and adhesive otitis media

Risks

- Significant complications are rare
- Infection, chronic otitis media, may occur as an immediate or late complication
- The ear may discharge continuously if there is a chronic cholesterol granuloma involving the mastoid or middle ear

- Tympanosclerosis, white patches of the tympanic membrane is believed by some to occur more commonly following the insertion of a ventilation tube
- The lumen of the ventilation tube may become blocked by dried blood of inspissated effusion
- A keratin foreign-body granuloma may develop around the ventilation tube, a tube granuloma
- A ventilation tube may be dropped through the myringotomy incision and become "lost" in the middle ear
- A persistent perforation may develop at the site where the ventilation tube was inserted. This occurs most commonly following the extrusion of wide, diameter-long stay ventilation tubes, e.g., "T tubes"
- Extremely rarely, damage may occur to the middle-ear ossicles, to a high jugular bulb, to a dehiscent facial nerve or to an ectopic carotid artery that passes through the middle ear

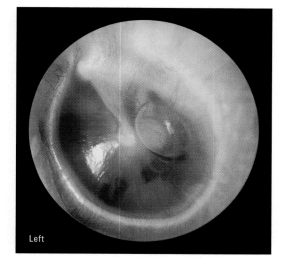

Left

Figure 6.1 Serous otitis media prior to myringotomy

A myringotomy is performed for a variety of reasons. This patient with serous otitis media was scheduled for a trans-Atlantic flight later in the day, and a myringotomy was indicated to prevent traumatic barotrauma. Note the air bubble in the posterior superior quadrant.

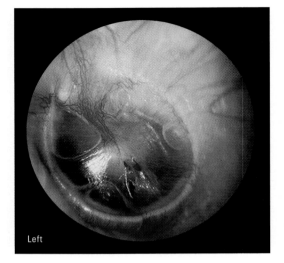

Left

Figure 6.2 Serous otitis media post myringotomy

This is the same patient ten minutes later. A small, vertical myringotomy incision has been made through the tympanic membrane in the six o'clock position, and the golden-yellow fluid within the middle ear has been aspirated. A few strands of fluid can be seen behind the tympanic membrane. Note the reflex vasodilatation of the malleolar vessels.

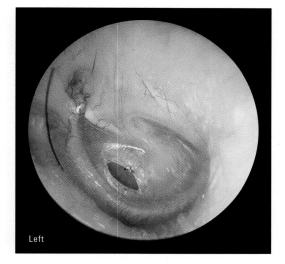

Left

Figure 6.3 Myringotomy incision

A medium-sized myringotomy incision can be seen in the seven o'clock position of this left tympanic membrane. Most myringotomy incisions heal spontaneously within seven to ten days.

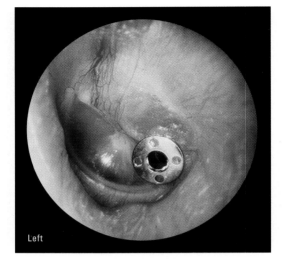

Left

Figure 6.4 Reutter bobbin ventilation tube

A stainless-steel Reutter bobbin tube, courtesy of Smith Nephew Richards, can be seen in the posteroinferior quadrant of this left tympanic membrane. This type of Reutter bobbin usually stays in place and functional for about 12 months.

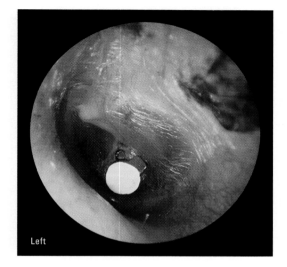

Left

Figure 6.5 Castelli semipermeable membrane tube

The lumen of this green Silastic ventilation tube is covered with a semipermeable membrane that allows the flow of gas for pressure equalization and prevents the ingress of water. This type of tube usually stays in place and functional for about 6 to 10 months.

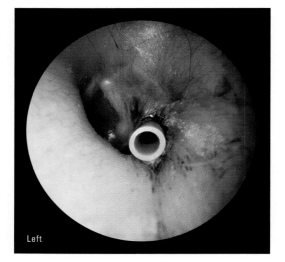

Left

Figure 6.6 Long-term T tube
A light-blue large-bore T tube has been inserted through the posterior inferior quadrant of
this left tympanic membrane. This type of
large-bore T tube usually stays in place and
functional for about 1 to 2 years.

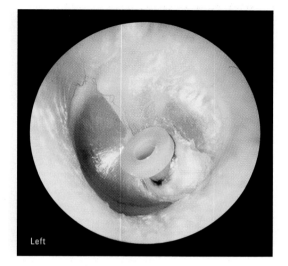

Left

Figure 6.7 Extruding tube

After a variable period of time, most tubes are gradually extruded by the tympanic membrane. Note the large collar of keratin that appears to be lifting this green Silastic ventilation tube out of the drum.

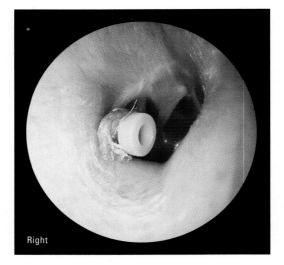

Right

Figure 6.8 Extruded tube

This brilliant-green Silastic bobbin-type tube
has been extruded by the tympanic membrane
and is slowly being carried laterally by the
normal migratory activity of the skin lining
the external canal.

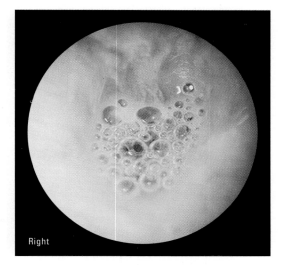

Right

Figure 6.9 Otitis media draining through a ventilation tube

Note the mixture of air bubbles and mucopurulent discharge in the deep canal. The hole in the tube allows the egress of pus directly from the middle ear. In this situation, a sample of the discharge should be taken for culture and sensitivity studies.

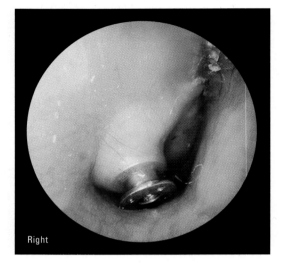

Right

Figure 6.10 Otitis media in an ear with a blocked ventilation tube

When the lumen of a tube is blocked, the tube is unable to perform any of its functions. This young girl has developed an acute otitis media. The discharge in the middle ear cannot flow out the blocked lumen and, instead, the entire stainless-steel Reutter bobbin is being pushed out of the tympanic membrane.

....

7

TUBE GRANULOMA

Definition

- The development of a localized mass of granulation tissue in the area adjacent to the shaft of a ventilation tube
- The mass of granulation tissue can be quite exuberant in some cases

Incidence

- An uncommon complication of ventilation-tube insertion
- Occurs in 0.5 to 1 percent of patients

Pathogenesis

- Some of the keratin squames around the base of the ventilation tube become implanted in the epidermis
- Keratin squames are considered to be a foreign protein, a foreign body
- The result is the development of a granulation tissue reaction to the keratin
- This is a true keratin foreign-body granuloma

Symptoms

- A painless, profuse otorrhea caused by

weeping from the infected and unepithelial-
ized surface of the granulation tissue
• Possible blood tingeing of the discharge, or
even a spontaneous, painless bloody discharge
from the ear canal

Otoscopic Appearance

• Otoscopic appearance varies from a small and
insignificant nubbin of friable granulation
tissue adjacent to the base of the tube or protruding from its lumen, to a large, polypoid
mass of granulation tissue that surrounds,
and in some cases even engulfs the tube
• In some cases, the granulation tissue may
become large enough to block the external
auditory canal

Treatment

• Removal of the tube
• Removal of the granulation tissue from its
site of attachment to the lateral surface of the
tympanic membrane
• The use of a suitable, topical antibiotic and
steroid eardrop during the healing process

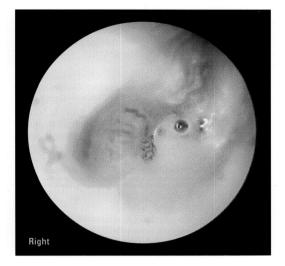

Right

Figure 7.1 Tube granuloma
This patient, in whose right ear a stainless-
steel Reutter bobbin had been inserted one
year previously, presented with a painless
otorrhea. Note the creamy-yellow, purulent
discharge in the deep canal and the bright-
pink vascular mass seen on the posterior half
of the eardrum.

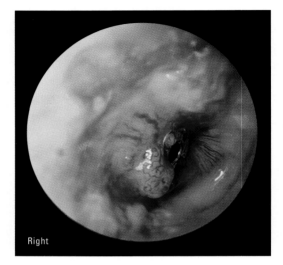

Right

Figure 7.2 Tube granuloma
After microdebridement of the discharge, the stainless-steel Reutter bobbin can be seen surrounded by the mass of granulation tissue.

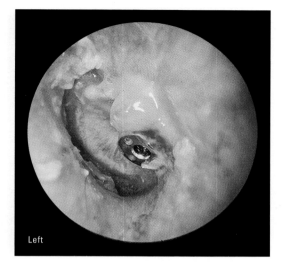

Left

Figure 7.3 Tube granuloma

A small tube granuloma can be seen arising from the lateral surface of the tympanic membrane just above the stainless-steel ventilation tube.

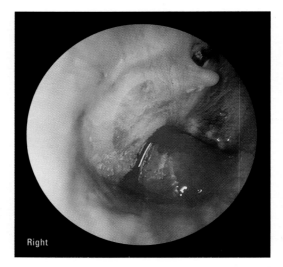

Right

Figure 7.4 Tube granuloma
A tube granuloma can be very vascular and
may be misdiagnosed as a vascular tumor.
This moderate tube granuloma was originally
believed to be a glomus tumor.

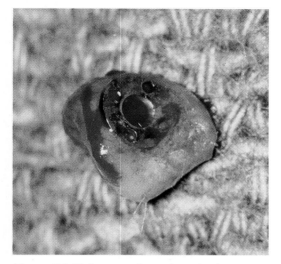

Figure 7.5 Tube granuloma (surgical specimen)

A tube granuloma is readily treated by the removal of the tube, with the adjacent granulation tissue, from the tympanic membrane. Note how the granulation tissue has completely surrounded the stainless-steel Reutter bobbin.

8

....

ATELECTASIS OF THE MIDDLE EAR

- Middle-ear atelectasis is the result of chronic eustachian-tube obstruction
- Atelectasis is characterized by atrophic changes in the fibrous middle layer of the drum, and by a partial or complete retraction of the tympanic membrane
- In atelectasis, the tympanic membrane does not adhere to the medial wall of the middle ear, and thus the process is reversible if the middle ear can be re-aerated
- Re-aeration of the middle ear is most easily re-established through inserting a ventilation tube

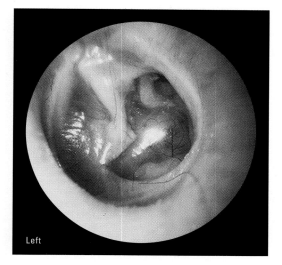

Left

Figure 8.1 Retraction pocket

The posterior half of this left tympanic membrane is atrophic and retracted medially. The result is a large retraction pocket. Note the golden-yellow, serous transudate filling the middle ear.

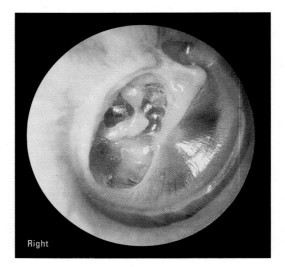

Right

Figure 8.2 Retraction pocket with ossicular erosion

This large, posterior retraction pocket lies directly on top of the head of the stapes, a condition that is termed "a natural myringost-apediopexy." Note how the end of the long process has been eroded, with only a fibrous band attaching the incus to the stapes. The middle ear is aerated.

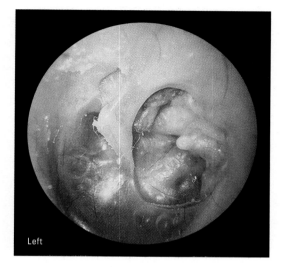

Left

Figure 8.3 Large, non-self-cleaning retraction pocket

The large, posterior retraction pocket of this left tympanic membrane has lost its self-cleansing ability. The result is an accumulation of keratin debris within the pocket. This type of retraction pocket can develop into a cholesteatoma.

9

ADHESIVE OTITIS MEDIA

- Adhesive otitis media is the end result of severe and recurrent middle-ear infections and atelectasis
- Like middle-ear atelectasis, adhesive otitis media is characterized by atrophic changes and a partial or complete retraction of the tympanic membrane toward the medial wall of the middle ear
- In adhesive otitis media, the difference is that the tympanic membrane is bound to the medial wall of the middle ear by numerous, fibrous adhesions
- Consequently, the retraction of the tympanic membrane cannot be reversed by re-aeration of the middle ear
- Adhesive otitis media is, thus, an end-stage condition and is essentially irreversible

Stages of Atelectasis

1 Retracted ear
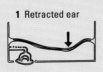

2 Severe retraction
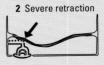

3 Atelectasis
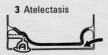

4 Adhesive otitis
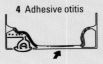

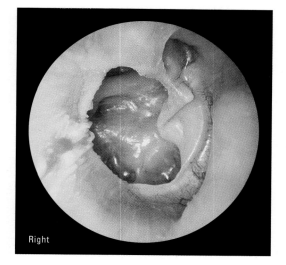

Right

Figure 9.1 Adhesive otitis media

The large, posterior retraction pocket in this right tympanic membrane has become "stuck" to the medial wall of the middle ear by numerous fibrous adhesions. This irreversible condition is known as "adhesive otitis media."

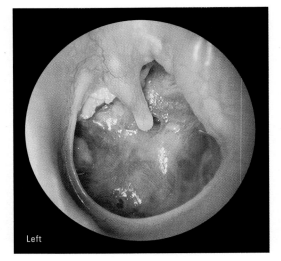

Left

Figure 9.2 Severe, adhesive otitis media

The entire tympanic membrane in this patient has become retracted onto the medial wall of the middle ear, where it is fixed by adhesions. At first glance, it appeared that this patient had a large, subtotal perforation of the tympanic membrane. On closer inspection, it became apparent that the tympanic membrane was thin and atrophic and "plastered" onto the medial wall of the middle ear. Note the collection of white keratin squame debris under the anterior bony annulus, which suggests the possibility of a cholesteatoma.

10

CHOLESTEATOMA

- Infrequent but serious complication of Eustachian-tube dysfunction
- Eustachian-tube dysfunction causes middle-ear atelectasis
- If a non-self-cleaning retraction pocket forms, keratin squame debris will accumulate within the retraction pocket
- Accumulating keratin debris causes the retraction pocket to enlarge
- Retraction pocket expands into the middle ear and mastoid; it erodes the adjacent bony structures, i.e., the ossicles and the bony walls of the mastoid
- Observation of white keratin debris within a retraction pocket or within a perforation strongly suggests the presence of a cholesteatoma

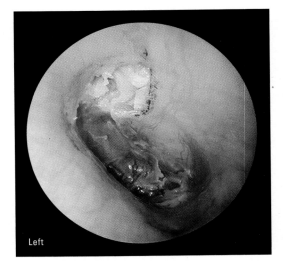

Left

Figure 10.1 Attic cholesteatoma

The collection of white keratin debris in this large, attic retraction pocket is characteristic of a cholesteatoma. Note the white mass of the cholesteatoma descending behind the tympanic membrane posteriorly.

11

ANTIBOTIC TREATMENT

ACUTE OTITIS MEDIA

Newborns

- Suggest using the same initial therapy as recommended for older adults
- Amoxicillin with potassium clavulanate
  (40 mg/kg/day PO divided into three doses
  Q 8 H), *or*
- Cefaclor
  (40 mg/kg/day PO divided into three doses
  Q 8 H)
- May have an advantage, because of their increased activity, against coliforms and *Staphylococci*, which cause 10 to 20 percent of these cases
- If no clinical improvement, a sample of the middle-ear fluid should be obtained for culture via tympanocentesis

Infants and Children

- Amoxicillin
  (40 mg/kg/day PO divided into three doses
  Q 8 H), *or*
- Amoxicillin with potassium clavulanate
  (40 mg/kg/day PO divided into three doses
  Q 8 H), *or*

- Cefaclor
  (40 mg/kg/day PO divided into three doses
  Q 8 H), *or*
- Erythromycin-sulfa combination
  (Erythromycin component 40 mg/kg/day PO
  divided into four doses Q 6 H), *or*
- Trimethoprim/sulfamethoxazole
  (6 to 8 mg/kg/day of the TMP component PO
  divided into two doses Q 12 hours, *or*
  Cefixime 8 mg/kg/day once daily *or* divided
  into two doses Q 12 hours
- If the tympanic membrane has ruptured, a
  sample of any discharge should be taken for
  gram stain and culture
- If there has been prior antibiotic therapy, or
  an immunocompromised host, one should
  suspect the presence of an unusual pathogen,
  and a sample of the middle-ear fluid should
  be obtained for culture by tympanocentesis

Reference

Nelson JD. 1991-1992 Pocketbook of
Pediatric Antimicrobial Therapy, 9th ed.
Williams & Wilkins, Baltimore MD, 1991.

ACUTE OTITIS MEDIA 2

Amoxicillin

Advantages

- Inexpensive
- Well tolerated
- Safe
- Drug of choice for more than 20 years
- Good activity against *Streptococcus pneumoniae*
- Activity against nonresistant *Haemophilus influenzae*

Disadvantages

- Contraindicated in penicillin-sensitive individuals
- Occasional patient will develop diarrhea
- Occasional patient will develop skin rash
- Not effective against Beta-lactamase, producing strains of *Haemophilus influenzae* (16 percent) and *Moraxella catarrhali* (80 percent)

Amoxicillin and Clavulanic Acid

Advantages

- Broad spectrum of antimicrobial activity
- Very effective against Beta-lactamase producing strains of *Haemophilus influenzae* and *Moraxella catarrhalis*

- Q 8 H dosing
- Generally well tolerated

Disadvantages

- Contraindicated in penicillin-sensitive individuals
- Occasional patient will develop diarrhea
- Occasional patient will develop skin rash
- More expensive than amoxicillin alone

Cefaclor

Advantages

- Good antimicrobial activity against the four major pathogens
- b.i.d. *or* t.i.d. dosing
- Safe
- Generally well tolerated

Disadvantages

- Contraindicated in penicillin-sensitive individuals
- Occasional serum sickness-like reaction
- More expensive than amoxicillin alone

Cefiximine

Advantages

- Good antimicrobial activity against the four major pathogens
- b.i.d. dosing

Disadvantages

- Contraindicated in penicillin-sensitive individuals
- Significant number of patients will develop gastrointestinal side effects
- Poor coverage against *Staphylococci*

Erythromycin / Sulfisoxazole

Advantages

- Good antimicrobial activity against the four major pathogens
- b.i.d. dosing

Disadvantages

- Contraindicated in infants less than two months old
- Contraindicated in sulfa-sensitive individuals
- Significant number of patients will develop gastrointestinal side effects
- Significant number of patients will develop dermatologic side effects

Trimethoprim / Sulfamethoxazole

Advantages

- Good antimicrobial activity against the four major pathogens
- Inexpensive
- b.i.d. dosing

Disadvantages

- Contraindicated in sulpha-sensitive individuals
- Coverage against group A *Streptococci*
- Allergic reactions to sulfamethoxazole can be severe, and in rare cases, fatal reactions have occurred: Stevens-Johnson Syndrome, fulminant hepatic necrosis, agranulocytosis, aplastic anaemia and epidermal necrolysis

GLOSSARY

Asymptomatic otitis media: a middle-ear effusion that was not present at a previous visit in a patient without fever or irritability

Chronic otitis media: a middle-ear effusion that lasts three months or longer

Effusion: a collection of relatively thick fluid in the middle ear. Effusions may be mucoid or purulent.

Middle-ear cleft: The middle ear cleft consists of four normally air-filled, interconnected structures: the Eustachian tube; the middle ear; the aditus ad antrum, which connects the middle ear to the mastoid; and the mastoid air cell system.

Mucoid effusion: the thick, opalescent, mucoid effusion present in the middle ear in patients with mucoid otitis media

Myringotomy: an incision through the tympanic membrane. A myringotomy is usually performed to allow access to the middle ear for the aspiration of the middle-ear contents for either diagnostic or therapeutic purposes.

Otitis media: a broad generic term that refers to an inflammatory process that affects the entire middle-ear cleft.

Otitis prone child: any child who has had at least six episodes of acute otitis media before six years of age. The otitis-prone child develops, with almost every upper-respiratory infection, a purulent middle-ear infection requiring antibiotic treatment. These children have a greater frequency of colonization of the nasopharynx by *Haemophilus influenzae*.

Otorrhea: discharge through a perforation in the tympanic membrane

Recurrent otitis media: three or more episodes of otitis media

Serous transudate: the thin, clear, golden-yellow fluid found in the middle ear in patients with serous otitis media

Tympanocentesis: trans-tympanic needle aspiration of the middle ear. Tympanocentesis is performed to obtain a sample of middle-ear fluid for microbiologic study

Tympanostomy: the insertion of a ventilation tube through the tympanic membrane

INDEX

Note: *t* indicates table, *f* indicates figure

Acute otitis media, *see also* other categories of Otitis
    media,vi*t*, 1-48, 65, 69
  Effusion, 12, 32*f*, 33*f*, 40*f*
  Epidemiology, 1-3
  Histopathology, 13
  Incidence, 2*f*, 3
  Microbiology, 7-9, 8*f*, 9*f*
  Pathogenesis, 5-9
    adenoids, 6-7, 16, 17, 43*f*
    Eustachian tube, 6
  Persistent, 16
  Recurrent, 16-17
    prevention of, 17
  Risk factors, 3-5
  Stages of, 9-12
    Eustachian-tube obstruction, 10, 28*f*
    redness, 10, 29*f*
    resolution, 12, 34*f*, 37*f*, 38f, 39*f*
    suppuration, 10-12, 30*f*, 33*f*
  Symptoms, 1
  Treatment, 13-16
Adenoids, 47*f*, *see also* other categories of Otitis
    media
  Hypertrophy, 45*f*, 46*f*, 47*f*
  Nasal mucosa changes, 44*f*
  Pathogenesis
    facies, 43f
Adhesive otitis media, 122-124
  Atelectasis, 123*f*, 124*f*
  Keratin, 124*f*
  Stages, 122
Air-Fluid level, 39*f*, 92*f*, 93*f*
Antibiotics, 12, 13-17, 39*f*, 69-70, 127-132, *see also*
    individual antibiotics and Treatments
  Treatment

    children, 15-16, 127-128
    infants, 15-16, 127-128
    newborns, 15, 127
    older adults, 15, 127
Amoxicillin, 15, 127, 129
  and Clavulanic acid, 129-130
  with Potassium clavulanate, 15, 127
Atelectasis, *see also* Adhesive otitis media of middle
    ear, 118-121, 119*f*, 120*f*, 121

Bullous myringitis, 41*f*, 42*f see also* Adhesive otitis
    media

Casts, 49-56, *see also* Tympanic membrane
  Histopathology, 51
Cefaclor, 15, 127, 128, 130
Cefixime, 128, 130-131
Cholesteatoma, 125-126, 126*f*
  Congenital, 26*f*, 27*f*
  Potential, 121*f*, 124*f*
Crusts, 49-56, *see also* Tympanic membrane
  Histopathology, 51

Effusion, *see also* categories of Otitis media, 12
  Persistence, 73*f*
Erythromycin-sulfisoxazole, 15, 128, 131

Mastoiditis, 57-63, 60*f*, 61*f*, 62*f*, 63*f*
  Diagnosis, 59
    differential, 58
  Etiology, 57
  Symptoms, 58
  Treatment, 59
Mucoid otitis media, vit, 64-82, 75*f*, 76*f*, 77*f*, 78*f*
    see also other categories of Otitis media
  Adenoids, 72
  Diagnosis, differential, 88*f*
  Effusion, 67-68, 70-72, 79*f*, 80*f*
    histology, 81*f*
    persistence, 73
  Epidemiology, 64
  Histology, 82*f*
  Histopathology, 72

Microbiology, 66-68, 68*t*
Pathophysiology, 69-70
Predisposing factors, 64-66
Sequelae, 74
Symptoms, 70-72
Synonyms, 64
Treatment, 72-73
Myringotomy, 13, 72, 97, 102*f*, 103*f*, *see also*
    Perforation entries
Indications, 97, 101*f*
Nature's, 12

Otitis media, *see also* categories of Otitis media, vi,
    vi*t*, 20*f*

Serous otitis media, vi*t*, 83-96, 89*f*, 90*f*, 91*f*
Adenoids, 85
Causes, 85, 96*f*
Diagnosis, 96*f*
    differential, 88*t*
Effusion, 85, 86, 94*f*
    histology, 95*f*
Epidemiology, 83
Histopathology, 86
hydrops ex vacuo, 84
Pathophysiology, 83-84
Symptoms, 85
Treatment, 87

Tonsils, 72
Hypertrophy, 48*f*
Trimethoprim/sulfamethoxazole, 15, 128, 131-132
Tube granuloma, 111-117, 113*f*, 114*f*, 115*f*, 116*f*,
    117*f*
Incidence, 111
Pathogenesis, 111
Symptoms, 111-112
Treatment, 112
Turbinates, 44*f*
Tympanic membrane, *see also* Atelectasis, categories
    of Otitis media, and Ventilation tubes
Casts, 49, 51, 53*f*, 54*f*, 55*f*, 56*f*
Crusts, 50, 51, 52*f*

Infection, 10-12, 31*f*, 32*f*, 35*f*, 36*f*
Keratin, 11, 23*f*, 24f, 25*f*, 36*f*, 121*f*, 124*f*, 125*f*,
      126*f*
Migrating ink dots, 21*f*, 22*f*
Normal, 18*f*, 19*f*, 54*f*
Perforation of, 11-12, 13, 32*f*, 34*f*, 37*f*, 38*f*, 70
Prominent vascular strip, 20*f*
Tympanocentesis, 15, 97
Indications, 97, 127, 128
Tympanostomy, 97-98
Indications, 99
Risks, 99-100, 110*f*, 111-117
Tubes, *see also* Ventilation tubes, 17
      blocked, 110*f*
      design, 98
      function, 98, 109*f*, 110*f*
      granuloma, 111-117
      names, 98

Vascular strip, on tympanic membrane, 20*f*
Ventilation tubes, *see also* Tympanostomy and Tube
      granuloma, 98, 104*f*, 105*f*, 106*f*
Extruding, 107*f*, 108*f*